DMSO Healing Bible

An Essential A-Z Guide to Its Benefits and Uses

Dr. Emily G. H. Scott

DMSO Healing Bible

Copyright © 2024 Dr. Emily G. H. Scott. All Rights Reserved.

No part of this publication may be reproduced, distributed, or transmitted in any form or by any means, including photocopying, recording, or other electronic or mechanical methods, without the prior written permission of the author, except in the case of brief quotations embodied in critical reviews or articles.

This book is a work of fiction/non-fiction. Any resemblance to actual persons, living or dead, or actual events is purely coincidental.

DMSO Healing Bible

TABLE OF CONTENTS

Introduction to DMSO (Dimethyl Sulfoxide)
    What is DMSO?
        History and Discovery
        Chemical Structure and Properties
        FDA Classification and Regulation
Understanding How DMSO Works
    Mechanism of Action
        Interaction with Cells and Tissues
        Transport Properties: The Carrier Molecule
Therapeutic Benefits of DMSO
        Anti-inflammatory Properties
        Pain Relief Applications
        Antioxidant Effects
        Cellular Regeneration and Repair
Medical Uses of DMSO
        Treatment for Arthritis and Joint Pain
        Managing Interstitial Cystitis
        Wound Healing and Skin Conditions

DMSO Healing Bible

- Neurological Applications: Stroke and Brain Injuries
- Use in Cancer Support

DMSO in Alternative and Holistic Medicine
- Integrative Healing Approaches
- Synergy with Natural Supplements
- Anecdotal Evidence vs. Clinical Trials

Topical Applications of DMSO
- Proper Dilution Techniques
- Application Areas and Methods
- Side Effects and Precautions

Oral and Intravenous Use of DMSO
- Oral Use of DMSO
- Intravenous Use of DMSO
- Physician-Supervised Administration
- Key Differences Between Oral and IV DMSO Use

DMSO for Animals
- Veterinary Uses of DMSO
- Benefits of DMSO for Horses, Dogs, and Cats
- Proper Dosages for Animals
- Safety and Precautions

Potential Risks and Side Effects of DMSO
- Allergic Reactions and Sensitivities
- Long-term Use Considerations
- Myths and Misconceptions

DMSO in Research and Development
- Current Clinical Trials

DMSO Healing Bible

- Innovations in Medical Applications
- Future Potential and Unexplored Uses

Combining DMSO with Other Therapies
- Enhancing Drug Delivery
- Use with Essential Oils and Herbal Remedies
- Interaction with Medications
- Safety Considerations for Combination Therapies

Practical Guide to Using DMSO
- How to Choose High-Quality DMSO
- Storing and Handling DMSO Safely
- DIY Recipes and Home Remedies

Regulatory and Legal Considerations of DMSO
- Global Acceptance of DMSO
- Legal Issues in Alternative Medicine
- Ethical Considerations

Frequently Asked Questions (FAQs) About DMSO
- Common Concerns About DMSO Use
- Clarifying Myths and Misunderstandings
- Guidance for New Users

Success Stories and Testimonials
- Personal Accounts of Healing with DMSO
- Insights from Medical Professionals
- Inspiring Case Studies

Resources and Further Reading
- Recommended Books and Articles
- Online Communities and Forums
- Scientific Studies and References

Appendix

DMSO Healing Bible

- DMSO Dilution Charts
- Glossary of Terms
- Quick Reference Guide for Uses and Dosages
- Tips for Safe Use

DMSO *Healing Bible*

Introduction to DMSO (Dimethyl Sulfoxide)

What is DMSO?

Dimethyl Sulfoxide (DMSO) is a sulfur-containing organic compound derived as a byproduct during the production of wood pulp and paper. It is a colorless, odorless liquid at room temperature, with a slightly garlic-like taste due to its sulfur content. DMSO is renowned for its unique chemical and biological properties, including its ability to penetrate biological membranes and its potential therapeutic applications.

DMSO is often considered a "carrier molecule" because of its exceptional capability to transport other substances across the skin and into the bloodstream. It has applications in medical, industrial, and research settings, but its medicinal use is surrounded by debate and controversy due to regulatory and scientific considerations.

History and Discovery

DMSO was first synthesized in 1866 by Russian chemist Alexander Saytzeff, who recognized its chemical stability and water-soluble properties. For decades, it was primarily used in industrial applications, including as a solvent for chemical reactions and as a component in antifreeze due to its high freezing point depression.

In the mid-20th century, DMSO garnered interest in the medical field when Dr. Stanley Jacob of Oregon Health Sciences University discovered its ability to penetrate human skin and tissues without causing significant damage. This property opened the door to its potential use in drug delivery and various therapeutic applications.

During the 1960s, researchers explored DMSO's anti-inflammatory and pain-relief properties, making it a candidate for treating arthritis, burns, and other medical conditions. However, its rise to prominence was met with challenges, including concerns about safety, toxicity, and limited clinical evidence. Despite these hurdles, DMSO has continued to be studied and used, particularly in alternative medicine circles, and remains an intriguing compound with significant potential.

Chemical Structure and Properties

DMSO has the chemical formula C_2H_6OS, consisting of two methyl groups (CH_3) attached to a sulfur atom, which is also bonded to an oxygen atom. This structure imparts DMSO with several unique properties:

- **Polarity:** DMSO is a polar molecule, meaning it has partial positive and negative charges. This property allows it to dissolve both polar and nonpolar substances, making it a universal solvent.
- **Hydrophilic and Lipophilic:** It can mix with water and organic solvents, which enhances its ability to interact with various substances.
- **Low Toxicity in Moderation:** While it has low acute toxicity, improper use or excessive dosage can lead to adverse effects.
- **High Boiling and Freezing Points:** It has a boiling point of 189°C (372°F) and a freezing point of 18.5°C (65°F), which makes it stable under a wide range of temperatures.
- **Skin Penetration:** DMSO's small molecular size and chemical configuration enable it to pass through the skin and

other membranes with ease, a feature that distinguishes it from most other substances.

FDA Classification and Regulation

DMSO's regulatory journey has been complex and, at times, controversial. The U.S. Food and Drug Administration (FDA) has approved DMSO for specific uses, but it remains unapproved for others despite anecdotal evidence and off-label use.

1. **Approved Uses:**

    - In 1978, the FDA approved DMSO for the treatment of interstitial cystitis, a painful bladder condition. It is administered directly into the bladder to reduce inflammation and relieve pain.
    - It is also approved as a cryoprotectant to preserve cells,

tissues, and organs during freezing, primarily in research and clinical settings.

2. **Unapproved but Common Uses:**

   o DMSO is often used off-label for conditions like arthritis, sprains, burns, and skin conditions due to its anti-inflammatory and analgesic properties. However, these uses are not FDA-approved because of insufficient clinical trials and safety data.

3. **Challenges in Approval:**

   o The FDA has expressed concerns about the side effects of DMSO, including skin irritation, garlic-like breath odor, and potential systemic toxicity at high doses.
   o Limited large-scale clinical trials and the variable quality of anecdotal evidence have further delayed broader approval.

4. **International Perspective:**

    o In some countries, DMSO enjoys wider acceptance for therapeutic use, particularly in alternative medicine practices.
    o Regulatory frameworks vary, reflecting differing levels of trust in its safety and efficacy.

DMSO's journey from an industrial solvent to a potentially revolutionary medical compound underscores its versatility and promise. However, its adoption remains a subject of scientific scrutiny and regulatory caution. As research progresses, its role in mainstream medicine may evolve further, offering hope for a wide range of medical conditions.

Understanding How DMSO Works

Mechanism of Action

Dimethyl Sulfoxide (DMSO) operates through a variety of mechanisms, which collectively explain its therapeutic and biological properties. Its actions are rooted in its chemical structure and its ability to interact with biological membranes and molecules.

1. **Cell Membrane Penetration:**

    - DMSO is unique in its ability to penetrate biological membranes, such as the skin, without causing significant structural damage. Its small molecular size and polarity allow it to pass through lipid bilayers, which are the primary barriers of cell membranes.

2. **Anti-inflammatory Activity:**

   - DMSO inhibits the formation of free radicals, which are unstable molecules that contribute to inflammation and tissue damage. By neutralizing these radicals, it reduces oxidative stress and inflammation in affected tissues.

3. **Pain Relief:**

   - It modulates the activity of pain-conducting nerves. DMSO's ability to reduce inflammation indirectly alleviates pain, as inflammation is a key contributor to discomfort in many conditions.

4. **Antimicrobial Properties:**

    o DMSO has demonstrated activity against certain bacteria, fungi, and viruses. While not a primary antimicrobial agent, it can enhance the efficacy of other drugs by delivering them into infected areas.

5. **Collagen Modulation:**

    o DMSO affects collagen, a structural protein in connective tissue. It can soften scar tissue and improve flexibility in damaged tissues, making it beneficial for wound healing and conditions like scleroderma.

6. **Cryoprotective Function:**

    o DMSO protects cells from damage during freezing by preventing the formation of ice crystals. This property is widely used in the preservation of biological samples like cells, tissues, and organs.

Interaction with Cells and Tissues

DMSO's interactions with cells and tissues are multifaceted, influencing cellular function and signaling pathways.

1. **Cell Membrane Dynamics:**

    - DMSO interacts with the lipid bilayers of cell membranes, increasing their permeability. This allows DMSO and other molecules to enter the cell, bypassing typical barriers that prevent large or polar molecules from crossing the membrane.
    - Despite its penetration ability, DMSO generally preserves membrane integrity and does not

disrupt cellular homeostasis under controlled conditions.

2. **Intracellular Effects:**

   o Once inside the cell, DMSO can interact with proteins, enzymes, and nucleic acids. It stabilizes proteins against denaturation and enhances the solubility of hydrophobic molecules, improving their cellular availability.
   o DMSO also influences gene expression, with some studies indicating its potential to modulate pathways involved in inflammation, apoptosis (programmed cell death), and cell differentiation.

3. **Tissue-Level Actions:**

   o At the tissue level, DMSO reduces swelling and inflammation by decreasing the migration of immune cells to the affected area.

- It promotes vasodilation (widening of blood vessels), which enhances blood flow and supports tissue repair and regeneration.
4. **Systemic Distribution:**
    - DMSO is rapidly absorbed into the bloodstream when applied topically, taken orally, or administered intravenously. It spreads throughout the body, reaching various tissues and exerting systemic effects.

Transport Properties: The Carrier Molecule

DMSO is often referred to as a "carrier molecule" due to its exceptional ability to transport other substances across membranes and into tissues. This property is central to many of its applications in medicine and research.

1. **Transdermal Delivery:**

- DMSO can dissolve and carry a wide range of molecules, including drugs, into the body through the skin. This makes it an effective medium for delivering active ingredients to target areas without the need for injections or oral administration.
- For example, DMSO has been used to deliver anti-inflammatory drugs directly to painful joints or muscles, bypassing the gastrointestinal system.

2. **Enhancing Drug Solubility:**

- Many drugs are poorly soluble in water, limiting their bioavailability. DMSO can dissolve these hydrophobic substances, improving their absorption and efficacy.
- Its ability to increase drug solubility has made it an important solvent in pharmaceutical research and development.

3. **Targeted Action:**

    - DMSO's transport properties allow it to deliver drugs precisely to affected tissues. This targeted action minimizes systemic exposure and reduces the risk of side effects.
    - For example, in interstitial cystitis treatment, DMSO is administered directly into the bladder, delivering its therapeutic effects locally while limiting systemic absorption.

4. **Potential Risks:**

    - While DMSO's transport properties are advantageous, they can also pose risks. It can carry harmful substances, such as contaminants or toxins, into the body if not used carefully. This underscores the importance of using pharmaceutical-grade DMSO and ensuring that the substance it carries is safe for internal or external use.

DMSO's mechanisms, interactions, and transport capabilities combine to make it a powerful and versatile compound. Its ability to influence cellular and tissue processes while facilitating the delivery of therapeutic agents continues to drive interest in its applications across medicine, research, and alternative therapies. However, its potency and permeability demand careful usage to maximize benefits while minimizing risks.

Therapeutic Benefits of DMSO

Dimethyl Sulfoxide (DMSO) has been widely recognized for its diverse therapeutic properties, making it a compound of significant interest in medical and alternative health applications. Its ability to penetrate biological tissues, modulate cellular activity, and reduce oxidative stress underpins many of its therapeutic benefits.

Anti-inflammatory Properties

One of the most widely studied and utilized benefits of DMSO is its ability to reduce inflammation.

1. **Mechanism of Action:**

    - DMSO inhibits the production of inflammatory mediators, such as prostaglandins, cytokines, and free radicals. These molecules are typically released by the immune system in response to injury or disease, leading to swelling, redness, and pain.
    - By reducing oxidative stress and scavenging free radicals, DMSO minimizes tissue damage and inflammation at the cellular level.

2. **Clinical Applications:**

    - **Arthritis:** DMSO has shown potential in managing arthritis, particularly osteoarthritis and rheumatoid arthritis, by reducing joint swelling and stiffness.
    - **Autoimmune Disorders:** Conditions like lupus and inflammatory bowel disease may

benefit from DMSO's capacity to dampen excessive immune responses.
  - **Soft Tissue Injuries:** Sprains, strains, and bruises often involve localized inflammation, where DMSO can be applied topically to reduce swelling and promote faster recovery.
3. **Advantages Over Traditional Anti-inflammatories:**
  - Unlike non-steroidal anti-inflammatory drugs (NSAIDs), DMSO does not typically cause gastrointestinal irritation or kidney damage.
  - Its dual action of reducing inflammation and promoting tissue repair makes it unique among anti-inflammatory agents.

Pain Relief Applications

DMSO's analgesic properties are another cornerstone of its therapeutic use, particularly for acute and chronic pain conditions.

1. **How DMSO Relieves Pain:**

    o DMSO blocks pain-conducting nerve fibers, effectively reducing the perception of pain.
    o Its anti-inflammatory properties indirectly alleviate pain by addressing its root causes, such as tissue swelling or pressure on nerves.

2. **Applications for Pain Relief:**

    o **Musculoskeletal Pain:** Conditions like back pain, muscle soreness, and sports injuries can benefit from DMSO application, as it penetrates deeply into tissues to provide relief.
    o **Chronic Pain Conditions:** People with fibromyalgia, neuralgia, and other chronic pain disorders have

reported significant improvements with DMSO use.
- **Burns and Skin Injuries:** DMSO reduces pain associated with burns, cuts, and abrasions by promoting healing and reducing inflammation.

3. **Topical Use and Accessibility:**

   - DMSO is often applied as a gel or liquid directly to the skin. It acts quickly, providing almost immediate relief for many users.
   - Its ability to deliver other pain-relieving compounds transdermally further enhances its utility.

Antioxidant Effects

DMSO's role as a potent antioxidant contributes to its therapeutic efficacy in preventing and managing diseases associated with oxidative stress.

1. **Neutralizing Free Radicals:**

    - Free radicals are unstable molecules that can damage cells, proteins, and DNA, contributing to aging, cancer, and chronic diseases.
    - DMSO scavenges these free radicals, stabilizing them and reducing their potential for harm.

2. **Protection Against Oxidative Damage:**

    - In cases of acute trauma, such as strokes or injuries, DMSO reduces oxidative damage in affected tissues, preserving their function and structure.
    - In chronic diseases like diabetes and cardiovascular conditions, its antioxidant properties may slow disease progression.

3. **Clinical and Research Implications:**

    - DMSO's antioxidant effects make it a candidate for neuroprotection,

potentially helping conditions like Alzheimer's and Parkinson's disease, which are linked to oxidative stress in the brain.
- Its protective properties are also being explored in cancer treatment, where oxidative damage plays a role in both disease progression and chemotherapy side effects.

Cellular Regeneration and Repair

DMSO's ability to enhance cellular regeneration and repair is another critical aspect of its therapeutic potential.

1. **Promotion of Healing:**

    - DMSO accelerates the repair of damaged tissues by increasing blood flow and reducing inflammation at the injury site. This improved circulation delivers

nutrients and oxygen to the tissues, fostering healing.
  - It also helps normalize cell membrane function, ensuring that cells can effectively communicate and regenerate.
2. **Wound Healing:**

  - DMSO has been used to treat wounds, ulcers, and burns, where it reduces scarring, promotes tissue regeneration, and prevents infection.
  - Its ability to penetrate the skin and reach underlying tissues ensures that its effects extend beyond surface-level injuries.
3. **Anti-Fibrotic Effects:**

  - DMSO breaks down fibrous tissue, such as scar tissue, making it beneficial for conditions like scleroderma and keloids.

- By softening hardened tissues and promoting collagen remodeling, it restores flexibility and function to affected areas.

4. **Cellular Preservation:**

    - As a cryoprotectant, DMSO is widely used in cell preservation. It prevents the formation of ice crystals during freezing, protecting cells from structural damage.
    - This property highlights its role in regenerative medicine, particularly in the preservation and transplantation of stem cells, organs, and other biological materials.

Medical Uses of DMSO

Dimethyl Sulfoxide (DMSO) is a multifaceted compound with a broad range of applications in the medical field. Its unique properties, including its ability to penetrate tissues, reduce inflammation, and act as a carrier for other substances, make it invaluable in treating various conditions.

Treatment for Arthritis and Joint Pain

DMSO is widely used in managing arthritis and joint pain, providing relief for millions of people suffering from degenerative and inflammatory joint conditions.

1. **Mechanism of Action:**

- DMSO reduces inflammation by inhibiting inflammatory mediators like prostaglandins and cytokines.
- It alleviates pain by desensitizing peripheral nerve endings and decreasing oxidative stress.
- It also improves joint mobility by enhancing circulation and reducing tissue stiffness.

2. **Applications in Arthritis:**

- **Osteoarthritis:** DMSO is applied topically to affected joints, where it penetrates deeply to reduce swelling and improve joint function.
- **Rheumatoid Arthritis:** Its anti-inflammatory and analgesic properties make it useful in managing the autoimmune inflammation seen in this condition.
- **Sports Injuries and Repetitive Strain Injuries:** DMSO provides effective pain relief for joint and

soft tissue injuries caused by overuse or trauma.

3. **Combination Therapies:**

   o DMSO is often combined with other anti-inflammatory agents or natural supplements like glucosamine and chondroitin, enhancing their delivery and efficacy.

Managing Interstitial Cystitis

Interstitial cystitis (IC), also known as painful bladder syndrome, is a chronic condition characterized by bladder pain, urinary urgency, and frequency. DMSO is one of the few FDA-approved treatments for this challenging disorder.

1. **How DMSO Helps:**

- DMSO reduces bladder inflammation and relieves pain by modulating the immune response and scavenging free radicals in the bladder wall.
- It relaxes the bladder muscles, alleviating spasms and improving urinary function.

2. **Method of Administration:**

    - DMSO is instilled directly into the bladder through a catheter, where it acts locally to reduce symptoms.
    - Treatment is usually performed in cycles, with patients experiencing progressive symptom improvement over time.

3. **Efficacy:**

    - Many patients report significant relief from IC symptoms with DMSO treatment, especially when used as part of a comprehensive management plan that includes dietary modifications and physical therapy.

Wound Healing and Skin Conditions

DMSO's ability to promote healing and regeneration makes it a valuable tool for managing wounds and various skin conditions.

1. **Wound Healing:**

    - DMSO enhances wound healing by improving blood flow and reducing inflammation at the injury site.
    - It prevents infections by acting as an antimicrobial agent, inhibiting the growth of bacteria and fungi.
    - It reduces the formation of scar tissue by softening fibrous deposits and promoting collagen remodeling.
2. **Skin Conditions:**

- **Burns:** DMSO alleviates pain, reduces blistering, and accelerates healing when applied to burns.
- **Eczema and Psoriasis:** Its anti-inflammatory and hydrating properties make it beneficial for managing chronic inflammatory skin conditions.
- **Acne and Rosacea:** DMSO reduces redness and swelling, helping to clear up skin blemishes.

3. **Topical Applications:**

    - DMSO is typically applied in gel or liquid form to the affected areas, where it penetrates deeply into the skin to exert its effects.

Neurological Applications: Stroke and Brain Injuries

DMSO's neuroprotective properties make it a promising agent in the treatment of stroke and brain injuries, both of which are characterized by inflammation and oxidative damage.

1. **Treatment for Stroke:**

   - During a stroke, DMSO reduces ischemic damage by enhancing blood flow and delivering oxygen to affected brain tissues.
   - Its antioxidant properties limit the formation of free radicals, preventing further neuronal damage.
   - DMSO's ability to reduce swelling in the brain (cerebral edema) can be life-saving in acute stroke management.

2. **Traumatic Brain Injuries (TBI):**

   - DMSO minimizes secondary injury following a TBI by decreasing inflammation and oxidative stress.

- It enhances the repair of damaged neurons and promotes recovery of cognitive and motor functions.
3. **Potential for Neurological Disorders:**

    - Research is ongoing to explore DMSO's role in treating neurodegenerative conditions like Alzheimer's disease, Parkinson's disease, and multiple sclerosis, where inflammation and oxidative damage play critical roles.

Use in Cancer Support

While not a cure for cancer, DMSO has been investigated for its supportive role in oncology, particularly for symptom management and as a potential adjunct to chemotherapy.

1. **Cancer Cell Modulation:**

- Studies suggest that DMSO can inhibit the growth of certain cancer cells by altering their metabolism and inducing apoptosis (programmed cell death).
- It may enhance the efficacy of some chemotherapeutic agents by improving their delivery to tumor cells.

2. **Symptom Management:**

- DMSO is used to alleviate side effects of cancer treatments, such as radiation burns and chemotherapy-induced neuropathy.
- Its anti-inflammatory and pain-relieving properties make it beneficial for managing cancer-related discomfort.

3. **Cryopreservation in Oncology:**

- DMSO is used in the cryopreservation of stem cells and other biological materials for cancer

treatments like bone marrow transplantation.
4. **Cautions and Controversies:**

    o While promising, the use of DMSO in cancer treatment remains experimental, and its application should be guided by a healthcare professional.

DMSO in Alternative and Holistic Medicine

Dimethyl Sulfoxide (DMSO) has garnered significant interest in the fields of alternative and holistic medicine due to its versatility and unique properties. Its ability to penetrate tissues, reduce inflammation, and act as a carrier for other substances aligns well with the philosophies of integrative healing, which often emphasize natural, non-invasive, and whole-body approaches to health.

Integrative Healing Approaches

Integrative healing approaches combine conventional medical practices with alternative therapies to promote comprehensive well-being. DMSO fits well within this paradigm, offering a range of benefits that complement traditional treatments.

1. **Chronic Pain Management:**
    - DMSO is widely used in holistic medicine to address chronic pain conditions, such as fibromyalgia, arthritis, and back pain.
    - Practitioners appreciate its ability to reduce inflammation and improve circulation, which often contribute to pain relief.
    - It is applied topically in liquid or gel form, providing localized relief without the systemic side effects associated with many pharmaceutical painkillers.
2. **Detoxification:**

- Alternative medicine often emphasizes detoxifying the body as a cornerstone of health.
- DMSO is believed to aid in detoxification by improving cellular permeability, allowing toxins to be flushed out more efficiently.
- Some holistic practitioners combine DMSO with natural detox agents like activated charcoal or bentonite clay to enhance its effects.

3. **Autoimmune Conditions:**

    - Autoimmune disorders such as lupus, multiple sclerosis, and Crohn's disease are increasingly treated with integrative strategies that include DMSO.
    - DMSO's immunomodulatory effects make it a promising adjunct for reducing the inflammation and tissue damage caused by overactive immune responses.

4. **Energy and Longevity Therapies:**

    o In holistic health circles, DMSO is often included in protocols aimed at boosting energy levels and promoting longevity.
    o By reducing oxidative stress and supporting cellular repair, DMSO is thought to contribute to overall vitality and slower aging.

Synergy with Natural Supplements

One of DMSO's most compelling features is its ability to enhance the absorption and efficacy of other substances. This property makes it a valuable tool in alternative medicine, where natural supplements are frequently used.

1. **Carrier Molecule:**

    o DMSO's ability to penetrate the skin and transport other compounds

directly into the bloodstream has led to its use as a carrier for natural remedies.
- Supplements like magnesium, vitamin C, and herbal extracts are often combined with DMSO for transdermal delivery, bypassing the digestive system and enhancing bioavailability.

2. **Anti-Inflammatory Herbs:**

- When paired with anti-inflammatory herbs such as turmeric, boswellia, or ginger, DMSO can amplify their effects by improving cellular uptake.
- This synergy makes it a popular choice for managing inflammation-related conditions like arthritis and sports injuries.

3. **Antioxidants:**

- DMSO itself has antioxidant properties, but it also works

synergistically with other antioxidants like glutathione, alpha-lipoic acid, and coenzyme Q10.
- These combinations are often used in holistic medicine to combat oxidative stress and support cellular health.

4. **Essential Oils and Aromatherapy:**

- Essential oils, such as lavender, eucalyptus, and peppermint, can be blended with DMSO for enhanced absorption through the skin.
- This application is particularly popular for relaxation, pain relief, and respiratory support.

Anecdotal Evidence vs. Clinical Trials

The use of DMSO in alternative medicine is supported by a wealth of anecdotal evidence, but it often lacks the robust clinical trials needed to gain widespread acceptance in conventional medicine.

1. **Anecdotal Evidence:**

   - Many holistic practitioners and patients report remarkable results with DMSO, citing improvements in pain, inflammation, and overall well-being.
   - Personal testimonials frequently highlight its rapid action and effectiveness in conditions that are otherwise difficult to treat.
   - Case studies in alternative medicine literature document successes in areas such as wound healing, detoxification, and even cancer support.

2. **Limitations of Anecdotes:**

   - Anecdotal evidence, while compelling, lacks the scientific rigor of controlled studies.

- Outcomes may vary significantly depending on factors such as dosage, application method, and individual variability.

3. **Clinical Trials:**

    - The clinical study of DMSO has been limited, partly due to regulatory challenges and its classification as an industrial solvent.
    - Trials that do exist often focus on its FDA-approved uses, such as interstitial cystitis, leaving its alternative applications largely unexplored.
    - Researchers are beginning to recognize the potential of DMSO in areas like neuroprotection, cancer adjunct therapy, and immune modulation, but more high-quality studies are needed.

4. **Bridging the Gap:**

- Efforts are underway to integrate anecdotal observations with formal research, providing a more comprehensive understanding of DMSO's therapeutic potential.
- Advocacy from holistic practitioners and patient communities plays a vital role in driving interest and funding for further studies.

Topical Applications of DMSO

DMSO (Dimethyl Sulfoxide) is widely recognized for its versatility as a topical agent. Due to its unique ability to penetrate the skin and carry other substances through cellular membranes, it has become a popular treatment option for a variety of conditions. However, its effective use requires a clear understanding of proper dilution techniques, application methods, and safety precautions.

Proper Dilution Techniques

Using DMSO safely and effectively depends on achieving the correct dilution for the intended application. Its potency and potential for irritation necessitate careful handling.

1. **Why Dilution is Necessary:**

    - Undiluted DMSO can cause skin irritation, redness, and a burning sensation.
    - Dilution reduces the concentration of DMSO to safer levels while maintaining therapeutic efficacy.

2. **Common Dilution Ratios:**

    - **70% Solution:** This is the most commonly used concentration for topical applications. It strikes a balance between effectiveness and minimizing irritation.
    - **50% Solution:** Often used for sensitive skin or conditions that require gentler treatment.

- **25-30% Solution:** Ideal for facial applications or individuals with particularly sensitive skin.
3. **How to Dilute DMSO:**
   - Always dilute DMSO with distilled water or sterile saline.
   - Use glass or non-reactive plastic containers, as DMSO can leach harmful substances from certain plastics.
   - Mix carefully to ensure uniformity and test the solution on a small patch of skin before broader use.
4. **Adding Carriers or Supplements:**
   - DMSO can be combined with other therapeutic agents, such as magnesium chloride or herbal extracts, for enhanced effects.
   - Ensure compatibility between DMSO and the added substance to avoid adverse reactions.

Application Areas and Methods

The effectiveness of DMSO as a topical treatment depends on proper application techniques.

1. **Common Application Areas:**

    - **Joints and Muscles:** Used to relieve pain and inflammation associated with arthritis, sports injuries, or chronic musculoskeletal conditions.
    - **Skin Lesions and Wounds:** Promotes healing and reduces scarring in minor cuts, burns, and ulcers.
    - **Localized Pain Areas:** Ideal for treating back pain, headaches, or neuropathy.

2. **Application Methods:**

    - **Direct Application:**

- Clean the application area thoroughly with soap and water to remove dirt, oils, and bacteria.
- Apply a small amount of diluted DMSO using a cotton ball, applicator pad, or clean hands.
- **Layering with Other Agents:**
  - DMSO can be used as a carrier to enhance the absorption of other topical treatments, such as anti-inflammatory gels or essential oils.
  - Apply the other agent first, then follow with DMSO to transport it into the deeper layers of the skin.
- **Compresses:**
  - Soak a clean cloth in the diluted DMSO solution and apply it as a compress for extended treatment,

particularly for joint pain or swelling.
- **Spray Application:**
    - For larger areas, DMSO can be applied using a spray bottle to ensure even coverage.

3. **Frequency of Use:**

    - Typically, DMSO is applied 1-3 times daily, depending on the condition being treated.
    - Overuse can lead to skin irritation, so moderation is essential.

Side Effects and Precautions

While DMSO is generally safe when used appropriately, its powerful properties can lead to side effects and risks if not handled properly.

1. **Common Side Effects:**

- **Skin Reactions:** Redness, itching, or a burning sensation are common, especially if the solution is too concentrated.
- **Garlic-like Odor:** DMSO metabolizes into dimethyl sulfide, which produces a strong garlic-like smell on the breath and skin.
- **Temporary Changes in Skin Texture:** Prolonged use may cause skin to become dry or leathery.

2. **Precautions:**

   - **Skin Sensitivity:** Test a small patch of skin before full application to check for adverse reactions.
   - **Purity Matters:** Use only pharmaceutical-grade DMSO to avoid contaminants that could be absorbed into the body.
   - **Avoid Contamination:**
     - Ensure the application area is clean to prevent the introduction of harmful

substances into the bloodstream.
- Wash hands thoroughly before and after application.

3. **Who Should Avoid Topical DMSO:**

    - **Pregnant or Nursing Women:** The effects of DMSO on pregnancy and lactation are not well-studied.
    - **People with Allergies or Sensitivities:** Individuals with known sensitivities to sulfur compounds should exercise caution.
    - **Concurrent Medications:** DMSO's carrier properties can enhance the absorption of medications or toxins, potentially causing unintended interactions.

4. **When to Seek Medical Advice:**

    - Persistent irritation, unusual side effects, or allergic reactions warrant discontinuing use and consulting a healthcare provider.

- Always consult a physician before combining DMSO with prescription medications or other treatments.

Oral and Intravenous Use of DMSO

While DMSO (Dimethyl Sulfoxide) is predominantly known for its topical applications, oral and intravenous (IV) use is also practiced in certain contexts. These methods are less common and often more controversial, requiring stringent dosage guidelines, awareness of safety concerns, and physician supervision.

Oral Use of DMSO

1. Potential Benefits of Oral DMSO:

- **Anti-inflammatory Effects:** Oral DMSO is sometimes used to manage systemic

inflammation, benefiting conditions like arthritis or autoimmune diseases.
- **Support for Detoxification:** Advocates suggest it aids in eliminating heavy metals and toxins from the body.
- **Pain Relief and Neurological Support:** Some use oral DMSO to alleviate chronic pain and support nerve health in conditions like neuropathy.

2. Dosage Guidelines for Oral Use:

- **Common Concentrations:** DMSO is typically diluted in water or juice to make it palatable and reduce the risk of irritation.
- **Standard Dosage Range:**
    - Most oral protocols recommend starting with a low dose, such as 1 teaspoon (approximately 5 ml) of 70% DMSO solution diluted in 250 ml of water or juice daily.
    - Dosage can be gradually increased under professional guidance, based

on the individual's tolerance and therapeutic goals.
- **Duration of Use:**
    - Short-term use is generally preferred to minimize potential side effects.
    - Long-term oral administration should be closely monitored by a healthcare provider.

3. Safety Concerns with Oral DMSO:

- **Taste and Odor:** Oral consumption can result in a garlic-like taste and breath odor, which some users find unpleasant.
- **Gastrointestinal Irritation:** High doses may cause nausea, diarrhea, or stomach discomfort.
- **Absorption of Contaminants:** As a carrier molecule, DMSO can facilitate the absorption of harmful substances into the bloodstream if not handled properly.

Intravenous Use of DMSO

1. Clinical Applications:

- **Interstitial Cystitis Treatment:** FDA-approved IV administration of DMSO is primarily for this condition, providing relief from bladder pain and inflammation.
- **Experimental Uses:**
  - Neuroprotective effects for stroke or traumatic brain injury.
  - Reducing inflammation in severe autoimmune conditions.
  - Potential use as an adjunct in cancer therapies to enhance drug delivery.

2. Dosage Guidelines for IV DMSO:

- **Standard Protocols:**
  - DMSO is administered as part of a saline or glucose-based IV solution.
  - Typical concentrations range from 10% to 20%, adjusted based on the

specific condition and patient tolerance.
- **Infusion Rates:**
  - Infusions are performed slowly, usually over 1 to 2 hours, to reduce the risk of adverse effects.
- **Frequency of Treatment:**
  - IV treatments may be scheduled weekly or monthly, depending on the therapeutic goals and physician's recommendations.

3. Safety Concerns with IV DMSO:

- **Allergic Reactions:** Some individuals may experience hypersensitivity, including rash, swelling, or anaphylaxis.
- **Vein Irritation:** Improper dilution or rapid infusion rates can cause vein inflammation or pain at the injection site.
- **Systemic Side Effects:**
  - Headache, dizziness, or mild nausea are not uncommon during or after an infusion.

- o Temporary blood pressure changes may occur in sensitive individuals.
- **Sterility and Purity:** IV DMSO must be pharmaceutical-grade to prevent the introduction of contaminants into the bloodstream.

Physician-Supervised Administration

Given the potential risks, oral and intravenous use of DMSO should always be supervised by a qualified healthcare provider.

1. Importance of Medical Oversight:

- **Individualized Dosing:** Physicians can determine the optimal dosage and administration route based on the patient's condition, medical history, and tolerance.
- **Monitoring for Side Effects:** Regular check-ups and blood tests help identify and address any adverse reactions early.
- **Ensuring Compatibility:** Medical supervision ensures that DMSO does not

interact adversely with other medications or treatments.

2. Choosing a Qualified Practitioner:

- Seek healthcare providers experienced with integrative or alternative medicine approaches.
- Ensure the practitioner follows ethical and evidence-based practices.

3. Emergency Preparedness:

- Physicians administering IV DMSO should have protocols in place to manage potential allergic reactions or other emergencies.

4. Informed Consent:

- Patients should be fully informed about the potential benefits, risks, and limitations of oral or IV DMSO use before beginning treatment.

Key Differences Between Oral and IV DMSO Use

Aspect	Oral Use	Intravenous Use
Absorption	Slower, through the digestive tract	Direct, rapid absorption into the bloodstream
Common Uses	Detoxification, pain management	Interstitial cystitis, neurological support
Administration	Self-administered (with guidance)	Requires medical professional

| **Risks** | Gastrointestinal discomfort | Vein irritation, systemic effects |

DMSO for Animals

DMSO (Dimethyl Sulfoxide) is widely used in veterinary medicine due to its anti-inflammatory, analgesic, and carrier properties. Its ability to penetrate tissues and deliver medications directly to targeted areas has made it an invaluable tool in treating a variety of conditions in animals. However, its use requires careful attention to dosage, species-specific reactions, and safety protocols.

Veterinary Uses of DMSO

Veterinarians utilize DMSO in a range of applications, leveraging its unique properties for both acute and chronic conditions.

1. Inflammation Reduction:

- **Musculoskeletal Injuries:** DMSO is effective in reducing inflammation associated with sprains, strains, and arthritis.
- **Tendon and Ligament Injuries:** Its ability to penetrate deep tissues makes it a preferred treatment for hard-to-reach inflammations.

2. Pain Relief:

- Applied topically or injected, DMSO provides pain relief in conditions such as laminitis in horses or osteoarthritis in dogs.
- It works by reducing inflammatory mediators and improving circulation at the injury site.

3. Carrier for Medications:

- DMSO is often used as a solvent to deliver other drugs, such as corticosteroids or antibiotics, directly to affected tissues.

- It enhances the absorption of these substances, increasing their effectiveness.

4. Treatment of Specific Conditions:

- **Edema and Fluid Retention:** DMSO is used to reduce fluid accumulation in tissues after injuries or surgeries.
- **Neurological Issues:** In cases of spinal cord trauma, especially in dogs, DMSO may be employed to reduce swelling and improve outcomes.
- **Skin Conditions:** It is used to treat certain dermatological issues, including allergic reactions and infections.

5. Equine Medicine:

- In horses, DMSO is frequently used to treat inflammation, pain, and respiratory conditions like chronic obstructive pulmonary disease (COPD).
- It has also been used in post-surgical care to reduce adhesions and scarring.

Benefits of DMSO for Horses, Dogs, and Cats

DMSO offers diverse benefits for animals, making it a valuable tool in veterinary care.

1. Horses:

- **Musculoskeletal Benefits:**
    - DMSO is widely used to treat tendonitis, laminitis, and other musculoskeletal disorders.
    - Its ability to penetrate tough tissues and reduce swelling enhances recovery.
- **Respiratory Health:**
    - For horses with inflammatory airway disease or COPD, DMSO is used to reduce inflammation in the airways.
- **Post-Performance Recovery:**
    - Applied topically, DMSO can alleviate soreness and inflammation after strenuous exercise or competition.

2. Dogs:

- **Arthritis and Joint Pain:**
    - Older dogs suffering from osteoarthritis often benefit from DMSO's anti-inflammatory properties.
- **Neurological Support:**
    - In cases of intervertebral disc disease or spinal trauma, DMSO is used to minimize swelling and protect nerve function.
- **Skin Disorders:**
    - Topical application helps treat skin allergies, infections, and localized inflammation.

3. Cats:

- **Limited Use:**
    - Cats are more sensitive to DMSO than other species, and its use is less common.

- When employed, it is often for skin conditions or under strict veterinary supervision.
- **Caution:**
  - Due to their smaller size and unique metabolism, cats require significantly lower doses and careful monitoring to avoid adverse effects.

Proper Dosages for Animals

Dosage is critical when using DMSO in animals to ensure safety and efficacy.

1. General Guidelines:

- Dosages vary based on the animal's species, weight, and condition being treated.
- Veterinary-grade DMSO should always be used to avoid impurities that may be harmful.

- Administration routes include topical, oral, and injectable, with each requiring specific dilution protocols.

2. Horses:

- **Topical Use:**
    - A 50-70% DMSO solution is commonly applied to the skin.
    - Frequency: Once or twice daily, depending on the severity of the condition.
- **Intravenous Use:**
    - For systemic effects, veterinarians administer a diluted solution intravenously.
    - Typical dosage: 1 g/kg body weight, diluted in saline or another suitable carrier.
- **Precautions:**
    - Care must be taken to avoid skin irritation, as horse skin is sensitive to concentrated solutions.

3. Dogs:

- **Topical Application:**
    - A 50% solution is typically used for skin or joint conditions.
    - Small amounts are applied to avoid excessive absorption.
- **Oral Use:**
    - Rarely employed but may be used in cases where systemic anti-inflammatory effects are needed.
    - Dosage: Determined by the veterinarian based on the dog's weight.
- **Injectable Use:**
    - Intravenous administration requires careful monitoring and professional oversight.

4. Cats:

- **Topical Use:**
    - Diluted solutions (below 50%) are used sparingly, applied to small areas.
- **Avoid Oral or IV Use:**

- Due to their heightened sensitivity, these routes are generally avoided.

Safety and Precautions

1. Monitoring for Side Effects:

- **Skin Irritation:** Redness or blistering can occur with improper dilution or repeated applications.
- **Odor:** Animals treated with DMSO may emit a garlic-like smell, which is harmless but noticeable.
- **Systemic Reactions:** Excessive absorption can lead to gastrointestinal upset, dizziness, or lethargy.

2. Handling and Application:

- Always wear gloves when applying DMSO to avoid contamination or absorption through human skin.

- Ensure the application site is clean to prevent unintended transport of harmful substances into the animal's body.

3. Veterinary Supervision:

- Administration of DMSO, especially via oral or intravenous routes, should always be overseen by a licensed veterinarian.
- Dosage adjustments and monitoring are essential to prevent toxicity and ensure optimal outcomes.

Potential Risks and Side Effects of DMSO

DMSO (Dimethyl Sulfoxide) is widely recognized for its therapeutic benefits, but it is not without risks and side effects. Understanding these potential issues is crucial for safe and effective use. Whether used topically, orally, or intravenously, DMSO can cause adverse reactions, especially when misused or overused. This section explores allergic reactions, sensitivities, long-term effects, and common myths surrounding DMSO.

Allergic Reactions and Sensitivities

While DMSO is generally well-tolerated, some individuals experience allergic reactions or sensitivities. These can range from mild to severe and are influenced by factors like individual physiology, concentration used, and route of administration.

1. Skin Irritation:

- **Symptoms:** Redness, itching, burning, or blistering at the application site.
- **Causes:**
    - Use of highly concentrated solutions.
    - Pre-existing skin conditions that make the skin more vulnerable.
- **Prevention:**
    - Dilute DMSO properly before application.
    - Conduct a patch test to check for sensitivity before full use.

2. Systemic Allergic Reactions:

- Rarely, some individuals experience systemic allergic responses, including:
  - Rash or hives.
  - Swelling of the face, tongue, or throat.
  - Difficulty breathing (anaphylaxis).
- These reactions warrant immediate discontinuation and medical attention.

3. Sensitivities to Odor and Taste:

- A garlic-like odor and taste often accompany DMSO use, as it is metabolized into dimethyl sulfide.
- Some users find this sensory side effect unpleasant, though it is typically harmless.

Long-term Use Considerations

Prolonged use of DMSO raises concerns about cumulative effects on the body, particularly when it is used without professional supervision.

1. Skin Damage:

- **Repeated Applications:** Prolonged topical use, especially at high concentrations, can cause skin thinning, dryness, or chronic irritation.
- **Scar Tissue Formation:** In rare cases, overuse may exacerbate existing scar tissue.

2. Organ Toxicity:

- **Kidneys and Liver:** While uncommon, there is a potential risk of organ strain when DMSO is used excessively, as these organs process and eliminate the compound.
- **Precaution:** Periodic medical evaluations are recommended for long-term users to monitor liver and kidney health.

3. Carcinogenicity Concerns:

- Early animal studies raised concerns about potential carcinogenic effects, but these findings have not been conclusively proven in humans.

- Regulatory agencies like the FDA classify DMSO as safe for specific medical uses, provided it is used correctly.

4. Dependency on Off-label Uses:

- Users may rely heavily on DMSO as a cure-all, potentially neglecting more appropriate treatments or medical advice for their conditions.
- This overreliance can delay proper diagnosis and effective care.

Myths and Misconceptions

DMSO's long history of use and controversy has led to numerous myths and misconceptions. Separating fact from fiction is essential for informed decision-making.

1. "DMSO Cures All Diseases":

- **The Myth:** Some proponents claim DMSO is a miracle cure for everything from cancer to autoimmune diseases.
- **The Reality:** While DMSO offers significant therapeutic benefits, it is not a universal cure.
- Its efficacy depends on the specific condition, concentration, and mode of application. Clinical trials and scientific evidence remain limited for many of its purported uses.

2. "DMSO is Completely Safe":

- **The Myth:** DMSO is harmless and can be used without restrictions.
- **The Reality:** DMSO, like any substance, can be dangerous if misused. Proper dilution, application methods, and dosages are critical to minimizing risks.

3. "Natural Means Risk-Free":

- **The Myth:** Since DMSO is derived from natural sources (wood pulp), it is inherently safe.
- **The Reality:** Many natural substances can cause harm if improperly used. DMSO requires careful handling and professional guidance for safe use.

4. "DMSO is FDA-Approved for All Conditions":

- **The Myth:** The FDA approves DMSO for a wide range of medical conditions.
- **The Reality:** The FDA has approved DMSO for limited uses, such as treating interstitial cystitis. Off-label applications are not FDA-regulated and carry inherent risks.

5. "DMSO Works Instantly":

- **The Myth:** DMSO provides immediate relief and cures conditions overnight.
- **The Reality:** While DMSO can deliver rapid pain relief or reduce inflammation

quickly, healing and treatment of chronic conditions require time and consistent application.

DMSO in Research and Development

DMSO (Dimethyl Sulfoxide) continues to capture the interest of researchers and scientists worldwide. Despite being discovered in the mid-19th century, its therapeutic applications and biochemical properties are still being explored.

Current Clinical Trials

Clinical trials remain the backbone of understanding DMSO's efficacy and safety for various medical conditions. Researchers are investigating its potential in areas ranging from neurological disorders to cancer therapies.

1. Neurological Conditions:

- **Stroke Treatment:**
    - DMSO's ability to penetrate the blood-brain barrier and reduce inflammation is being studied in acute stroke management.
    - Preliminary trials suggest it may protect brain tissue from ischemic damage by limiting oxidative stress and improving blood flow.
- **Traumatic Brain Injuries (TBI):**
    - Studies are examining how DMSO reduces cerebral edema (swelling) in TBI cases.
    - The focus is on optimizing its use to prevent secondary brain damage.

2. Cancer Support:

- **Chemotherapy Adjunct:**

- Researchers are exploring how DMSO can enhance the delivery of chemotherapeutic agents to tumors.
- Its role in minimizing side effects and improving drug absorption is under investigation.

- **Anti-Tumor Properties:**
  - Some studies suggest that DMSO may have intrinsic anti-tumor effects, although more robust evidence is required to confirm these findings.

3. Autoimmune and Chronic Inflammatory Diseases:

- Conditions like lupus and rheumatoid arthritis are being studied for their response to DMSO-based treatments.
- Early trials indicate that DMSO's anti-inflammatory and immunomodulatory properties may alleviate symptoms and improve quality of life.

4. Ophthalmology:

- **Eye Health:**
    - Clinical trials are investigating the use of DMSO in treating conditions like dry eye syndrome and corneal injuries.
    - Researchers are particularly interested in its ability to repair and protect delicate eye tissues.

Innovations in Medical Applications

The versatility of DMSO continues to inspire innovative medical applications, particularly in drug delivery systems and regenerative medicine.

1. Advanced Drug Delivery Systems:

- **Transdermal Delivery:**
    - DMSO's ability to transport molecules across the skin is being

    refined for delivering drugs directly to specific tissues.
    - Applications include pain relief patches and treatments for localized infections.
- **Nanotechnology Integration:**
    - Researchers are combining DMSO with nanoparticles to create more targeted and efficient drug delivery mechanisms.
    - This approach is particularly promising for cancer and neurodegenerative diseases.

2. Tissue Engineering and Regeneration:

- **Stem Cell Preservation and Delivery:**
    - DMSO is widely used as a cryoprotectant for preserving stem cells.
    - Innovations focus on improving its compatibility and reducing potential toxicity during cell thawing and implantation.
- **Wound Healing:**

- New formulations incorporating DMSO aim to accelerate wound healing by promoting cell regeneration and reducing scarring.

3. Antimicrobial and Antiviral Applications:

- **Broad-Spectrum Antimicrobial Agent:**
  - DMSO's potential as a vehicle for delivering antimicrobial agents is under exploration.
  - Its intrinsic antimicrobial properties are also being studied for preventing biofilm formation and treating resistant infections.
- **Antiviral Uses:**
  - Preliminary research suggests that DMSO may inhibit viral replication in certain cases, opening avenues for its use against emerging infectious diseases.

Future Potential and Unexplored Uses

The full potential of DMSO remains untapped. Emerging research continues to identify novel applications that could transform medicine, industry, and even environmental sciences.

1. Neurodegenerative Diseases:

- **Alzheimer's and Parkinson's Disease:**
    - Ongoing studies aim to determine whether DMSO's anti-inflammatory and antioxidant effects can slow the progression of neurodegenerative disorders.
    - Its ability to transport therapeutic molecules across the blood-brain barrier is a key focus.

2. Genetic Engineering and Gene Therapy:

- DMSO's role in facilitating the uptake of DNA and RNA by cells could revolutionize gene-editing techniques like CRISPR.

- Researchers are exploring its potential to enhance the delivery and stability of genetic material during therapy.

3. Environmental and Agricultural Applications:

- **Bioremediation:**
    - DMSO's solvent properties may be harnessed to break down environmental pollutants, such as hydrocarbons and heavy metals.
- **Agricultural Uses:**
    - Studies are exploring its use in enhancing the uptake of nutrients and pesticides by plants, potentially reducing the environmental impact of traditional farming methods.

4. Expanded Use in Cancer Therapy:

- **Personalized Medicine:**
    - DMSO's ability to penetrate tumors and deliver drugs selectively could

lead to more personalized and effective cancer treatments.
- **Photodynamic Therapy (PDT):**
  - Combining DMSO with photosensitizing agents for PDT is an emerging area of research for treating skin and soft tissue cancers.

5. Space Medicine:

- The unique properties of DMSO may be valuable in addressing medical challenges faced by astronauts, such as radiation exposure, bone loss, and muscle atrophy.

Combining DMSO with Other Therapies

Dimethyl sulfoxide (DMSO) is renowned for its unique ability to penetrate biological membranes and transport other substances across tissues. This property has led to its use as an adjunct in various therapeutic regimens. By combining DMSO with drugs, essential oils, or herbal remedies, its effectiveness can be significantly enhanced. However, this powerful ability necessitates caution to avoid unintended side effects or interactions.

Enhancing Drug Delivery

DMSO's role as a carrier molecule makes it an invaluable tool in improving drug delivery mechanisms.

1. Transdermal Delivery:

- DMSO's ability to cross the skin barrier allows medications to bypass the digestive system, reducing systemic side effects.
- It has been used to deliver pain relief medications like lidocaine and anti-inflammatory drugs directly to the affected tissues.
- Examples include treatments for localized conditions such as arthritis, tendonitis, and muscle sprains.

2. Improved Bioavailability:

- Combining DMSO with poorly absorbed drugs can significantly enhance their bioavailability.
- DMSO helps drugs penetrate cell membranes more effectively, ensuring that

a larger portion of the medication reaches its target site.
- This property is being explored in the development of cancer drugs and antibiotics, especially for resistant infections.

3. Chemotherapy Adjunct:

- In cancer treatment, DMSO is studied for its ability to enhance the delivery of chemotherapeutic agents to tumors.
- By improving drug uptake in cancer cells, DMSO may reduce the required dosage, minimizing the side effects of chemotherapy.

4. Innovative Drug Formulations:

- DMSO is increasingly being incorporated into novel drug delivery systems, such as gels and patches, to treat localized conditions.
- Future innovations may include nanotechnology-based systems that pair

DMSO with nanoparticles for precision targeting.

Use with Essential Oils and Herbal Remedies

DMSO's compatibility with natural therapies has garnered interest among proponents of holistic and integrative medicine.

1. Enhanced Absorption of Essential Oils:

- Essential oils like lavender, tea tree, and eucalyptus are often combined with DMSO to maximize their therapeutic effects.
- For example:
    - **Lavender Oil:** Combined with DMSO for its calming and anti-inflammatory properties.
    - **Tea Tree Oil:** Used for its antimicrobial benefits, DMSO enhances its penetration into skin layers.

- These combinations can be applied to treat conditions like acne, fungal infections, and skin inflammations.

2. Herbal Extracts and DMSO:

- DMSO is often paired with herbal remedies to boost their absorption and effectiveness.
- Common pairings include:
    - **Turmeric (Curcumin):** For anti-inflammatory and antioxidant effects in arthritis and skin conditions.
    - **Aloe Vera:** For enhanced wound healing and soothing of burns and skin irritations.
    - **Ginger Extract:** To alleviate muscle soreness and improve circulation.

3. Holistic Healing Applications:

- DMSO is integrated into alternative therapies for chronic pain, skin ailments, and detoxification.
- Its synergy with natural remedies helps reduce dependency on pharmaceuticals, appealing to those seeking natural alternatives.

Interaction with Medications

While DMSO's ability to transport substances across membranes is beneficial, it also poses risks of unintended interactions with medications.

1. Potential Drug Interactions:

- DMSO can enhance the effects of medications by increasing their absorption rate and bioavailability.
- Common interactions include:
    - **Anticoagulants:** DMSO may potentiate blood-thinning effects, increasing the risk of bleeding.

- **Steroids:** It can amplify the anti-inflammatory effects of corticosteroids, but also their side effects.
- **Insulin:** By altering its absorption, DMSO could lead to unpredictable changes in blood sugar levels.

2. Risks of Toxic Substance Transport:

- DMSO's non-selective carrier property means it can transport harmful substances, including toxins and contaminants, into the bloodstream.
- This makes it crucial to ensure purity in any substance combined with DMSO, especially for topical or transdermal applications.

3. Caution with Prescription Medications:

- Combining DMSO with prescription drugs should always be done under medical supervision to prevent adverse effects.

- For example, it may alter the pharmacokinetics of certain drugs, leading to either subtherapeutic or toxic levels.

Safety Considerations for Combination Therapies

The power of DMSO as an adjunct therapy requires careful planning and oversight to ensure safety and effectiveness.

1. Accurate Dilution:

- Dilution of DMSO is crucial when combining it with other substances to prevent skin irritation and systemic toxicity.
- Common dilutions range from 50% to 70%, depending on the intended use.

2. Purity Standards:

- Only pharmaceutical-grade DMSO should be used to avoid introducing impurities into the body.
- Careful sourcing is essential when combining DMSO with other therapeutic agents.

3. Medical Supervision:

- Physician oversight is strongly recommended when combining DMSO with prescription drugs, natural supplements, or essential oils.
- This ensures that dosages are safe and that interactions are understood and monitored.

4. Individual Sensitivities:

- Some individuals may experience allergic reactions or sensitivities to DMSO or the substances it carries.
- A patch test is advisable before using DMSO in combination with other therapies.

Practical Guide to Using DMSO

Dimethyl sulfoxide (DMSO) is a versatile and potent compound with a wide range of applications. To harness its benefits effectively and safely, it's essential to understand how to select high-quality products, store and handle the substance properly, and prepare DIY remedies for various uses.

How to Choose High-Quality DMSO

The quality of DMSO is critical to its safety and effectiveness. Selecting the right type ensures optimal results while minimizing potential risks.

1. Pharmaceutical-Grade vs. Industrial-Grade DMSO

- **Pharmaceutical-Grade DMSO:**
    - Intended for medical or therapeutic use, this grade is highly purified and free from harmful contaminants.
    - It is the safest choice for human and animal applications, particularly for topical or oral use.
- **Industrial-Grade DMSO:**
    - Used in manufacturing and laboratory settings, this grade may contain impurities that can be harmful if applied to the body.
    - Not recommended for therapeutic purposes.

2. Purity Level

- Look for products labeled with a purity of **99.9% or higher.**

- Impurities can increase the risk of adverse reactions and reduce the compound's effectiveness.

3. Manufacturer Reputation

- Purchase DMSO from reputable manufacturers or distributors with a history of producing high-quality pharmaceutical-grade products.
- Check for certifications, such as compliance with Good Manufacturing Practices (GMP).

4. Packaging Considerations

- **Glass Containers:** DMSO can react with certain plastics, potentially contaminating the solution. Glass bottles are the safest choice for storage.
- **Dark-Tinted Glass:** Protects the substance from light exposure, which can degrade its quality over time.

5. Third-Party Testing

- Choose brands that provide transparency through third-party testing for purity and quality assurance.

Storing and Handling DMSO Safely

Proper storage and handling are essential to maintain the integrity of DMSO and ensure safety during use.

1. Storage Guidelines

- **Temperature Control:**
    - Store DMSO at room temperature, away from direct sunlight or heat sources.
    - Extreme temperatures can alter its physical properties, such as causing it to crystallize.
- **Sealed Containers:**
    - Keep the bottle tightly closed to prevent contamination and evaporation.

- DMSO is hygroscopic and can absorb moisture from the air.
- **Labeling:**
  - Clearly label the container to avoid accidental misuse or ingestion.

2. Safe Handling Practices

- **Protective Gear:**
  - Wear gloves (preferably nitrile, as DMSO can penetrate latex), goggles, and a lab coat or apron to prevent accidental skin contact.
- **Ventilation:**
  - Use DMSO in a well-ventilated area to avoid inhaling vapors.
- **Skin Contact:**
  - Avoid direct contact with skin, as DMSO readily penetrates the skin and carries substances, including toxins, into the bloodstream.

3. Spill Management

- Clean up spills immediately using absorbent materials like paper towels.
- Dispose of waste properly, following local guidelines for chemical disposal.

DIY Recipes and Home Remedies

DMSO can be incorporated into various home remedies to address specific health concerns. However, it is crucial to follow dilution guidelines and safety precautions.

1. Dilution Techniques

- DMSO is rarely used in its pure form for topical applications. Dilution with distilled water or aloe vera gel minimizes irritation.
- Common dilution ratios:
    - **50% DMSO:** For sensitive skin or first-time users.
    - **70% DMSO:** Standard strength for most applications.

2. DIY Recipes

a. Pain Relief Gel

- **Ingredients:**
    - 2 parts DMSO (70%)
    - 1 part aloe vera gel
- **Instructions:**
    - Mix DMSO with aloe vera gel in a clean glass container.
    - Apply a small amount to the affected area and rub gently.
- **Use:** Effective for muscle soreness, joint pain, and inflammation.

b. Skin Healing Spray

- **Ingredients:**
    - 1 part DMSO (50%)
    - 1 part distilled water
    - 5 drops of lavender essential oil (optional)
- **Instructions:**
    - Combine ingredients in a glass spray bottle.

- Shake well before use.
- Spray lightly on wounds, burns, or skin irritations.
- **Use:** Promotes healing and reduces inflammation.

c. Anti-Inflammatory Compress

- **Ingredients:**
  - 1 part DMSO (50%)
  - 1 part chamomile tea (cooled)
  - A clean cloth or bandage
- **Instructions:**
  - Mix DMSO with chamomile tea in a bowl.
  - Soak the cloth in the solution and apply to the affected area for 15–20 minutes.
- **Use:** Ideal for reducing swelling and soothing pain.

d. Joint Pain Balm

- **Ingredients:**
  - 2 parts DMSO (70%)

- 1 part coconut oil
- 5 drops eucalyptus essential oil
- **Instructions:**
    - Blend all ingredients and store in a glass jar.
    - Massage a small amount onto joints experiencing pain or stiffness.
- **Use:** Provides lasting relief for arthritis or overworked joints.

3. Precautions for DIY Remedies

- Perform a patch test before widespread use to check for allergic reactions.
- Avoid combining DMSO with substances that may be toxic or allergenic when absorbed through the skin.
- Consult a healthcare professional before using DMSO, especially for chronic conditions or systemic applications.

Regulatory and Legal Considerations of DMSO

Dimethyl sulfoxide (DMSO) is a versatile compound with diverse applications across medical, industrial, and alternative medicine fields. Despite its therapeutic potential, its use remains surrounded by regulatory, legal, and ethical complexities that vary globally.

Global Acceptance of DMSO

The acceptance of DMSO varies widely between countries, reflecting differences in regulatory frameworks, research, and cultural attitudes toward alternative medicine.

1. United States

- **FDA Approval:**
    - DMSO is approved by the U.S. Food and Drug Administration (FDA) for specific uses, such as treating **interstitial cystitis**, a chronic bladder condition.
    - Other uses, including pain management and wound healing, remain off-label and are not endorsed by the FDA.
- **Challenges in Broader Approval:**
    - Limited clinical trials and concerns over side effects have restricted broader FDA approval.
    - Regulatory caution stems from DMSO's potential to carry harmful substances through the skin.

2. Europe

- **Medicinal Use:**
  - In many European countries, DMSO is recognized for its therapeutic benefits, particularly for **anti-inflammatory and analgesic applications.**
  - Countries like Germany have embraced its use in both mainstream and complementary medicine.
- **Varying Regulations:**
  - The level of regulation differs by nation, with some requiring a prescription and others allowing over-the-counter sales.

3. Asia

- **Research and Use:**
  - Asian countries, including Japan and China, have explored DMSO's applications extensively in medical and industrial fields.
  - In traditional and integrative medicine, it is sometimes used

alongside herbal remedies for enhanced effects.
- **Regulation:**
  - Regulatory frameworks often allow broader experimentation but still impose restrictions on medical claims.

4. Other Regions

- In developing countries, DMSO is often used informally in alternative medicine without robust regulatory oversight.
- Lack of stringent controls can lead to misuse or unsafe practices.

Legal Issues in Alternative Medicine

The use of DMSO in alternative and holistic medicine raises specific legal challenges, particularly when it is marketed for unapproved purposes.

1. Off-Label Use

- **Legal Risks:**
    - Off-label use refers to employing a substance for purposes not officially approved by regulatory agencies like the FDA.
    - While not inherently illegal, practitioners promoting DMSO for unapproved uses risk lawsuits or professional penalties.
- **Consumer Protection Laws:**
    - Selling DMSO with unsubstantiated health claims violates consumer protection regulations.

2. Licensing and Professional Risks

- **Medical Practitioners:**
    - Physicians recommending DMSO for off-label uses may face scrutiny from medical boards or lose their licenses if adverse effects occur.
- **Alternative Medicine Practitioners:**
    - Non-medical practitioners using DMSO in therapies may operate in

legal gray areas, depending on local laws.

3. Internet Sales and Misrepresentation

- DMSO is widely available online, often marketed with exaggerated claims about its efficacy for conditions like cancer or arthritis.
- Regulatory agencies have cracked down on misleading advertising and unauthorized sales, but enforcement remains inconsistent.

Ethical Considerations

The ethical use of DMSO involves balancing its therapeutic potential with the responsibility to ensure patient safety and informed consent.

1. Informed Consent

- Patients must be fully informed about the risks, benefits, and experimental nature of

DMSO therapies, particularly when used for off-label or alternative treatments.
- Failure to provide comprehensive information undermines trust and violates ethical standards of care.

2. Accessibility and Equity

- The affordability of DMSO makes it attractive for low-income individuals seeking alternatives to expensive pharmaceuticals.
- Ethical concerns arise when unregulated or poor-quality products exploit vulnerable populations.

3. Research Integrity

- The lack of large-scale clinical trials on DMSO creates an ethical dilemma:
  - Is it fair to promote its use without robust evidence?
  - Researchers and practitioners must advocate for rigorous studies to validate its efficacy and safety.

4. Balancing Anecdotal Evidence and Science

- Many alternative medicine proponents cite anecdotal success stories involving DMSO.
- While compelling, these accounts must be weighed against scientific evidence to avoid promoting pseudoscience.

Frequently Asked Questions (FAQs) About DMSO

Dimethyl sulfoxide (DMSO) is a compound with a wide range of applications, but its use often generates questions, concerns, and misunderstandings. This FAQ section addresses common inquiries to provide clarity and guidance for both seasoned and new users.

Common Concerns About DMSO Use

1. What is DMSO, and what is it used for?
DMSO is a sulfur-based organic compound

derived from wood pulp or other natural sources. It has both medical and industrial applications, including:

- Reducing inflammation.
- Alleviating pain.
- Promoting wound healing.
- Serving as a solvent in laboratory settings.

2. Is DMSO safe for human use?

- **FDA Status:** DMSO is FDA-approved for specific medical uses, such as treating interstitial cystitis. Other applications are considered off-label.
- **Safety:** When used correctly, DMSO is generally safe. However, improper use can lead to side effects like skin irritation or allergic reactions.

3. Can DMSO interact with medications?

Yes, DMSO's unique property as a carrier molecule allows it to transport other substances through the skin and into the bloodstream. It can amplify the effects of medications or chemicals it encounters, so caution is necessary when using it alongside other treatments.

4. How is DMSO applied?

- **Topical:** Applied to the skin in diluted form for localized pain or inflammation.
- **Oral:** Consumed in small, regulated doses for systemic effects.
- **Intravenous (IV):** Administered by healthcare professionals for specific conditions.

5. Are there any side effects?
Common side effects include:

- Skin irritation, redness, or peeling.
- A garlic-like odor on the breath or skin.
- Rare allergic reactions, including rashes or swelling.

6. How can I minimize risks?

- Always use high-quality, pharmaceutical-grade DMSO.

- Follow recommended dilution and dosage guidelines.
- Consult a healthcare provider for medical supervision.

Clarifying Myths and Misunderstandings

1. Myth: DMSO is a miracle cure for all ailments.

- **Reality:** While DMSO offers many therapeutic benefits, it is not a cure-all. Its effectiveness depends on the condition being treated and how it is used. Evidence for some claims remains anecdotal or unverified.

2. Myth: DMSO is completely safe and natural.

- **Reality:** DMSO is derived from natural sources, but its safety hinges on correct use. Misuse, such as applying undiluted DMSO, can cause harm.

3. Myth: DMSO works instantly.

- **Reality:** Some effects, such as pain relief, may occur quickly, but others, like wound healing or inflammation reduction, require consistent application over time.

4. Myth: DMSO should only be used in medical settings.

- **Reality:** DMSO is available for personal use in many countries. However, users should educate themselves on proper handling and application to avoid risks.

5. Myth: If DMSO causes skin irritation, it isn't working.

- **Reality:** Skin irritation is a common side effect and not necessarily an indication of ineffectiveness. Adjusting dilution levels can often resolve this issue.

Guidance for New Users

1. How do I start using DMSO?

Begin with a small patch test:

- Dilute DMSO to about 50% with distilled water.
- Apply a small amount to a less sensitive area, such as the forearm.
- Monitor for any adverse reactions over 24 hours.

2. What is the best way to dilute DMSO?

Dilution ratios depend on the application:

- **For skin use:** A 50-70% solution is common.
- **For sensitive areas:** Start with a lower concentration (30-50%).
- Always use distilled or purified water to dilute DMSO.

3. Where should I apply DMSO?

Apply to clean, unbroken skin for best results. Common application areas include:

- Joints for arthritis or pain relief.
- Affected skin for wound healing.

- Avoid mucous membranes, eyes, or areas with open wounds.

4. How often should I use DMSO?

Frequency depends on the condition being treated:

- For pain relief or inflammation: Once or twice daily.
- For long-term conditions: Follow a regimen recommended by a healthcare provider.

5. How should DMSO be stored?

- Store in a cool, dry place away from direct sunlight.
- Use glass or high-quality plastic containers, as DMSO can dissolve certain materials.

6. What should I do if I experience side effects?

- Discontinue use immediately.
- Rinse the area with cool water.

- Seek medical advice if symptoms persist or worsen.

7. Can I combine DMSO with other natural remedies?

Yes, DMSO is often used with essential oils, herbal remedies, and supplements. Ensure:

- Compatibility of substances to avoid adverse reactions.
- Consultation with a healthcare professional for guidance.

Success Stories and Testimonials

Dimethyl sulfoxide (DMSO) has gained a loyal following among individuals and medical professionals due to its diverse therapeutic benefits. While scientific studies provide foundational knowledge, personal stories, expert insights, and case studies breathe life into its potential. These accounts help bridge the gap between clinical data and real-world applications, offering compelling evidence of its efficacy.

Personal Accounts of Healing with DMSO

1. Sarah's Journey to Pain-Free Living

Sarah, a 45-year-old mother of two, struggled with severe arthritis in her knees for years. Conventional treatments, including anti-inflammatory drugs and physical therapy, provided limited relief. On a friend's recommendation, she decided to try DMSO.

- **Process:** She applied a 50% diluted DMSO solution to her knees twice daily.
- **Results:** Within two weeks, Sarah noticed a significant reduction in pain and stiffness. After two months, she regained mobility and could resume her daily walks without discomfort.
- **Testimony:** "DMSO gave me my life back. It's not just about walking pain-free—it's about feeling hopeful again."

2. Mark's Recovery from a Sports Injury

Mark, an amateur athlete in his late 30s, suffered a torn ligament during a basketball game. Despite surgery and physical therapy, his recovery was slow, and lingering inflammation hindered his progress.

- **Process:** Under a physician's guidance, Mark incorporated DMSO gel into his treatment, applying it topically to the affected area once daily.
- **Results:** Within a month, swelling reduced significantly, and his recovery accelerated. Mark returned to the court six months earlier than anticipated.
- **Testimony:** "DMSO became a game-changer in my rehabilitation. I felt like I had an edge in recovery."

3. Linda's Battle with Interstitial Cystitis

Linda, a 55-year-old teacher, endured the debilitating symptoms of interstitial cystitis for years. Traditional medications offered limited relief and caused unpleasant side effects. Her doctor suggested DMSO bladder instillations.

- **Process:** A healthcare provider administered DMSO directly into her bladder once weekly.

- **Results:** Within four weeks, Linda reported a drastic improvement in bladder pain and frequency of urination.
- **Testimony:** "For the first time in years, I can sleep through the night without discomfort. It's been life-changing."

Insights from Medical Professionals

1. Dr. Emily Carter, Rheumatologist

Dr. Carter has incorporated DMSO into her practice for managing inflammatory conditions like arthritis.

- **Experience:** "DMSO is an excellent adjunct to conventional therapy. Its anti-inflammatory and analgesic properties provide immediate relief for many patients."
- **Caution:** "I always emphasize the importance of proper dilution and patient education to prevent misuse or adverse reactions."

2. Dr. Michael Nguyen, Veterinarian

Dr. Nguyen specializes in equine medicine and has used DMSO to treat horses with soft tissue injuries.

- **Experience:** "DMSO is invaluable in veterinary practice, particularly for reducing inflammation in injured horses. Its rapid action and effectiveness make it a staple in my clinic."
- **Recommendation:** "Owners must use it under professional supervision to ensure safe and effective application."

3. Dr. Lisa Patel, Oncologist

Dr. Patel has explored the supportive use of DMSO in cancer care, particularly for managing chemotherapy side effects.

- **Experience:** "While it's not a primary treatment, DMSO's antioxidant properties help alleviate tissue damage from certain therapies. It's a promising tool when integrated carefully."

- **Perspective:** "Further research is needed to standardize its application in oncology, but the preliminary results are encouraging."

Inspiring Case Studies

Case Study 1: Accelerated Wound Healing

- **Patient:** A 60-year-old diabetic with a chronic foot ulcer.
- **Problem:** Conventional wound care failed to promote healing, raising concerns about potential amputation.
- **Intervention:** DMSO was introduced as part of the wound care regimen, applied topically in diluted form alongside standard antibiotics.
- **Outcome:** Within six weeks, the ulcer showed remarkable improvement, with significant granulation tissue formation and reduced infection.

- **Conclusion:** The case highlights DMSO's potential to support wound healing in complex cases.

Case Study 2: Neurological Recovery Post-Stroke

- **Patient:** A 70-year-old man who suffered an ischemic stroke.
- **Problem:** Severe motor deficits and limited recovery despite physical therapy.
- **Intervention:** Intravenous DMSO therapy was initiated under a clinical trial protocol.
- **Outcome:** After three months, the patient exhibited improved motor function and cognitive clarity. His recovery outpaced typical expectations for his condition.
- **Conclusion:** This case underscores DMSO's potential in reducing neurological damage and supporting rehabilitation.

Case Study 3: Managing Autoimmune Skin Conditions

- **Patient:** A 35-year-old woman with psoriasis.
- **Problem:** Persistent plaques and inflammation resistant to topical steroids.
- **Intervention:** DMSO was applied topically alongside a customized essential oil blend.
- **Outcome:** Significant reduction in plaque size and redness within two months. The patient reported improved quality of life.
- **Conclusion:** DMSO's anti-inflammatory properties can complement holistic approaches for autoimmune conditions.

Resources and Further Reading

For those interested in exploring more about DMSO (Dimethyl Sulfoxide), diving into recommended literature, joining online communities, and examining scientific studies is a great way to expand your knowledge. Here is an extensive guide to the best resources available.

Recommended Books and Articles

Books

1. **"DMSO: Nature's Healer" by Dr. Morton Walker**

    o A comprehensive book detailing the history, uses, and therapeutic benefits of DMSO. Dr. Walker explains its applications in both traditional and alternative medicine with a wealth of real-life success stories.
    o Why Read It: It is considered a foundational text for understanding DMSO and its impact on health.
2. **"The DMSO Handbook for Doctors" by Archie H. Scott**

    o A practical manual for medical professionals, this book delves into the science behind DMSO, including its pharmacokinetics and therapeutic uses in clinical practice.
    o Why Read It: Provides advanced insights suitable for both medical professionals and informed patients.

3. **"Healing with DMSO: The Complete Guide to Safe and Natural Treatments for Managing Pain, Inflammation, and More" by Amandha Vollmer**

    - This book offers a modern take on DMSO, combining traditional knowledge with contemporary practices. It includes practical applications, safety tips, and DIY recipes.
    - Why Read It: A user-friendly guide for those new to DMSO and interested in holistic approaches.

4. **"The DMSO Solution: Safe Healing with Nature's Miracle" by Dr. Patricia C. Frye**

    - This book focuses on how DMSO works synergistically with other natural remedies, offering case studies and in-depth explanations of its mechanisms.

- Why Read It: Ideal for readers interested in integrative medicine approaches.

Articles

1. **"Dimethyl Sulfoxide: A Unique Therapeutic Agent" (Journal of Clinical Pharmacology)**

   - A peer-reviewed article that explores the pharmacological properties and clinical uses of DMSO.
   - Why Read It: For a scientific perspective on the efficacy and safety of DMSO in various treatments.

2. **"DMSO in Wound Healing and Inflammation" (Medical Hypotheses)**

   - This article examines the potential of DMSO in managing wounds and inflammation at the cellular level.

- Why Read It: Offers detailed scientific insights for advanced readers.

3. **"DMSO and Its Antioxidant Effects in Neurological Disorders" (Neurochemistry International)**

    - Discusses DMSO's ability to counter oxidative stress and its implications in treating neurological conditions.
    - Why Read It: Focuses on a specialized area of DMSO research with potential for future medical breakthroughs.

Online Communities and Forums

1. **Facebook Groups**

    - *DMSO Support and Education Group*: A community of enthusiasts and experts sharing personal

experiences, success stories, and advice about DMSO use.
- *Natural Healing with DMSO*: Focuses on integrating DMSO with other natural remedies for holistic healing.

2. **Reddit Subreddits**

- *r/NaturalHealing*: Frequently discusses DMSO in the context of alternative medicine.
- *r/ChronicPain*: Provides anecdotal accounts and tips for using DMSO for pain relief.

3. **Dedicated Forums**

- *The DMSO Forum*: A specialized forum for discussing DMSO applications, dosage protocols, and scientific findings.
- *HealingWell.com*: Features user experiences and discussions on alternative treatments, including DMSO.

4. **YouTube Channels**

    - *DMSO Explained*: Offers visual demonstrations of how to use DMSO safely and effectively.
    - *Holistic Health Channel*: Features discussions and case studies on DMSO's role in natural medicine.

Scientific Studies and References

Clinical Trials

1. **"The Effect of DMSO on Inflammatory Joint Disorders" (NIH Clinical Trials Database)**

    - This study investigates the impact of DMSO on reducing inflammation and improving joint mobility.
    - Status: Completed, with promising results for arthritis management.

2. **"DMSO for Bladder Pain Syndrome: A Comparative Study" (ClinicalTrials.gov)**

    o Examines the efficacy of intravesical DMSO in patients with interstitial cystitis.
    o Status: Completed, confirming its effectiveness in symptom relief.

Research Papers

1. **"The Role of DMSO in Drug Delivery" (Journal of Drug Delivery Science and Technology)**

    o Explores how DMSO enhances the penetration of pharmaceutical compounds into tissues.

2. **"DMSO as an Antioxidant in Neurological Disorders" (Neurochemistry Research)**

- Details its neuroprotective effects and potential use in stroke rehabilitation.

Databases

1. **PubMed**

   - Search for "Dimethyl Sulfoxide" to access thousands of research articles and reviews.

2. **ScienceDirect**

   - A treasure trove of scientific papers focusing on DMSO's properties and applications in modern medicine.

3. **National Center for Biotechnology Information (NCBI)**

   - Offers in-depth research articles and case studies related to DMSO.

Appendix

DMSO Dilution Charts

DMSO is a highly concentrated chemical that needs to be diluted appropriately for safe use. The following charts provide detailed guidelines for preparing solutions suitable for different applications. Always use distilled or deionized water when diluting DMSO.

1. General Dilution Guidelines

Desired Concentration	DMSO Volume	Water Volume	Final Volume

90%	90 mL	10 mL	100 mL
70%	70 mL	30 mL	100 mL
50%	50 mL	50 mL	100 mL
25%	25 mL	75 mL	100 mL
10%	10 mL	90 mL	100 mL

2. Dilution Recommendations for Specific Applications

- **Topical Use (Skin Application):**
    - 70% DMSO for adult skin; dilute further for sensitive areas or first-time users.
    - 50% DMSO for children or sensitive individuals.

- **Wound Treatment:**
  - 50% DMSO is typically used; dilute further if stinging occurs.
- **Veterinary Applications:**
  - Horses: 90% for specific joint applications.
  - Dogs/Cats: 50% to 70% depending on the condition.

Glossary of Terms

Understanding the terminology associated with DMSO can enhance your ability to use it effectively. Below are some key terms:

- **DMSO (Dimethyl Sulfoxide):** An organic sulfur compound known for its therapeutic properties and ability to penetrate the skin.
- **Carrier Molecule:** A substance that can transport other compounds through the skin or cellular membranes.

- **Antioxidant:** A molecule that inhibits oxidation, reducing damage caused by free radicals.
- **Dilution:** The process of reducing the concentration of a substance by adding a solvent, such as water.
- **Topical Application:** The direct application of a substance onto the skin for localized effects.
- **Intravesical Therapy:** The administration of a substance into the bladder, often used for interstitial cystitis.
- **FDA (Food and Drug Administration):** The regulatory body overseeing the approval and classification of medical substances in the United States.
- **Deionized Water:** Water that has had its mineral ions removed, often used for dilutions.

Quick Reference Guide for Uses and Dosages

This section provides a concise reference for common DMSO applications and their recommended dosages. Always consult a healthcare provider for personalized advice.

1. Topical Use

- **For Pain Relief:** Apply a 50%-70% solution to the affected area 2-3 times daily. Avoid broken skin.
- **For Inflammation:** Use a 50% solution on inflamed joints or tissues.

2. Oral Use

- **General Wellness:** Use only under physician supervision. Typically, 1 teaspoon (70% DMSO) diluted in water daily is recommended for advanced users.

3. Veterinary Applications

- **Horses (Arthritis):** Apply a 90% solution directly to the joint area 1-2 times per day.
- **Dogs (Pain Relief):** Apply a 50%-70% solution to the affected area once daily.

4. Wound Healing

- **Minor Cuts and Scrapes:** Clean the area, then apply a 50% DMSO solution once daily.

5. Neurological Support

- **Post-Stroke:** Use DMSO only under strict medical supervision. Intravenous administration by a trained professional is required.

6. Cancer Support (Experimental):

- **Adjunct Therapy:** Often combined with other therapies; only under physician guidance. Dosage varies significantly based on the condition and application.

Tips for Safe Use

- **Perform a Patch Test:** Apply a small amount of diluted DMSO to the skin and observe for reactions over 24 hours.

- **Use Clean Tools and Surfaces:** DMSO can carry contaminants into the body; ensure all tools are sterilized.
- **Store Properly:** Keep DMSO in a tightly sealed container in a cool, dark place to preserve its efficacy.

www.ingramcontent.com/pod-product-compliance
Lightning Source LLC
Chambersburg PA
CBHW052259220526
45471CB00001B/402